KETOGENIC DIET

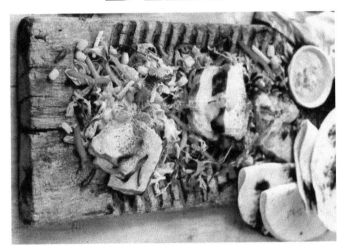

SALADS AND PORK COOKBOOK

Felicity Flinn

Table of Contents

SALADS

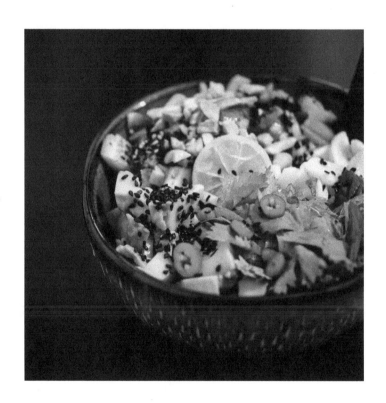

Chopped Hoagie Bowl (Keto)

(Ready in about 15 mins | Serving 8| Difficulty: Easy)

Per serving: Kcal: 421, Fat: 35g, Net Carbs: 3g, Protein: 21g

Ingredients

Bowl

- Chopped Roast turkey 8 oz

- Chopped Genoa salami 8 oz

- Chopped Smoked deli ham 8 oz

- Chopped Provolone cheese 8 oz

- Chopped cheddar cheese mild 4 oz

- Shredded Lettuce 3.5 oz

- Grape tomatoes 5&1/3 oz

- Cucumber, chopped & peeled 7 oz

- Banana peppers pickled, chopped rings 3 oz

- Red onion, diced 1/4

Sauce

- Mayonnaise ¾ c

- Vinegar Red wine ¼ c

- Olive oil 2 tbsp

- Dried basil 1 tsp

- Seasoning Italian ½ tsp

- Oregano dried 1 tsp

Instructions

- ❖ Put all the ingredients in the bowl in a large serving bowl & set aside.
- ❖ Whisk all of the sauce ingredients together in a separate bowl.
- ❖ Pour the sauce over meat, cheeses, and vegetables and combine to stir or toss.

Antipasto Salad

(Ready in about 15 mins | Serving 8| Difficulty: Easy)

Per serving: Kcal: 407, Fat: 35g, Carbs: 5g, Protein: 17g

Ingredients

- Romaine chopped 3 c

- Green olives halved 1/2 c

- Medium black olives 1/2 c

- Cherry tomatoes halved 1/2 c

- Mini pepperoni 1/2 c

- Jarred roasted chopped red peppers 1/4 c

- Genoa Salami 8 ounce

- Mozzarella cheese balls 1/2 c

- Artichoke hearts quartered 13 ounce

- Provolone cheese 8 ounces

Olive Oil Lemon Dressing:

- Olive oil 1/4 c

- lemon juice 1/2

- Italian seasoning 1 tsp

Instructions

- ❖ In a bid bowl add the olives, tomatoes, romaine, pepperoni, salami, mozzarella, red peppers, provolone, and artichoke hearts.
- ❖ Olive oil lemon dressing: In a bowl whisk the lemon juice, olive oil, & Italian seasoning. Pour the solid, then toss.

Low-Carb Eggplant Towers

(Ready in about 40 mins | Serving 4| Difficulty: Medium

Per serving: Kcal: 558, Fat: 49g, Net Carbs: 9g, Protein: 19g

Ingredients

- Fresh basil 8 oz
- Olive oil ½ c
- Balsamic vinegar 1.5 tbsp
- Garlic clove 1
- Salt ½ tsp
- Ground black pepper >>to taste
- Eggplant towers
- Eggplant 1
- Fresh mozzarella cheese log 9 oz
- Tomatoes 2
- Olive oil 2 tbsp

To serve

- Fresh basil 5 oz
- Cherry tomatoes 4 oz

Instructions

Basil dressing

❖ Place the basil, garlic, salt, as well as olive oil in a food processor for basil dressing and blend until smooth.

Eggplant towers

❖ Cut in ½ "(1 cm) slices of eggplant, mozzarella, and tomato.

❖ Heat the olive oil over medium heat in a frying pan & fry the eggplant until golden.

❖ Place an eggplant slice in the center of each plate to assemble the platter, then add a slice of mozzarella accompanied by a tomato slice.

❖ Add the basil dressing in a spoonful.

❖ Continue processing on single plates until all ingredients have been used, approximately 6 slices per tower.

❖ Complete your creations with a bit more basil dressing over the top and scatter some cherry tomatoes halves around the plate.

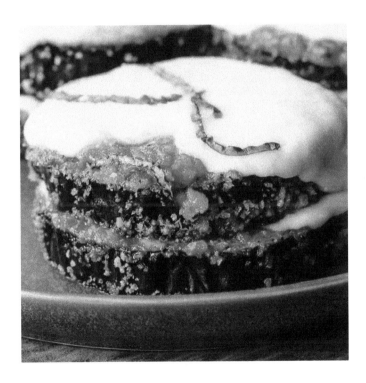

Shrimp Salad with Bacon Fat Dressing

(Ready in about 20 mins | Serving 4| Difficulty: Easy)

Per serving: Kcal: 455, Fat: 40g, Net Carbs: 2g, Protein: 21g

Ingredients

Spinach salad

- Fresh spinach 6 oz

- Bacon chopped 2 oz

- Hard-boiled eggs, chopped 2

- Shrimp, peeled & cleaned 1 lb.

- Ghee or butter 1 tbsp

- Parmesan cheese, grated 1 oz

Hot bacon fat dressing

- Bacon fat or light olive oil ½ c

- Apple cider vinegar ¼ c

- Dijon mustard 1 tbsp

- Salt>> to taste

- Ground black pepper>> to taste

Instructions

- ❖ Wash the spinach & remove stubborn ends. Dry the leaves. Divide the spinach equally between the plates.
- ❖ Fry the bacon at medium-high heat in a saucepan until crispy.
- ❖ Top spinach, divided evenly with hard-boiled eggs & bacon.
- ❖ With a towel, pat the shrimp to dry to remove as much extra water as possible. Melt the ghee in a large skillet over high heat. Throw the shrimp into the skillet & sauté for 3-5 minutes, until the shrimp is bright pink and cooked thoroughly.

- ❖ Split the shrimp into the plates, & sprinkle with Parmesan cheese.
- ❖ Heat the bacon fat using a small saucepan. In the apple cider vinegar, whisk together with the remaining ingredients. Serve warm & mix just before pouring.
- ❖ Dress up hot bacon fat vinaigrette salad dishes & serve immediately.

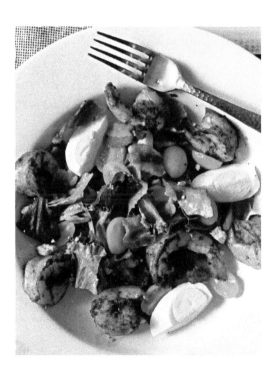

Cobb Refreshing Salad with Ranch Dressing – Keto

(Ready in about 35 mins | Serving 2| Difficulty: Easy)

Per serving: Kcal: 838, Fat: 63g, Net Carbs: 6g, Protein: 57g

Ingredients

Ranch dressing

- Mayonnaise 3 tbsp

- Ranch seasoning 1 tbsp

- Water 2 tbsp

- Eggs 2

- Bacon 3 oz

- Cut into pieces rotisserie chicken 1.5 lb.

- Blue cheese, crumbled 2 oz

- Avocado, sliced 1

- tomato, sliced 1

- Romaine lettuce, chopped 5 oz

- Fresh chives, minced 1 tbsp

- Salt & ground black pepper>> to taste

Instructions

- ❖ Begin with getting the dressing ready. Combine the mayonnaise, water and ranch seasoning. set it aside.
- ❖ Place in boiling water the eggs for 8 to 10 mins. For simplified peeling, cool in the ice water. Roughly chop them.
- ❖ In a hot skillet (dry) fry the bacon until crispy.
- ❖ Spread the lettuce with the chicken, vegetables, eggs, blue cheese, and bacon. Season with pepper and salt, the eggs especially.
- ❖ Drizzle with the dressing and finish with chives that have been finely chopped.

Keto Asian Beef Salad

(Ready in about 25 mins | Serving 2| Difficulty: Easy)

Per serving: Kcal: 1038, Fat: 96g, Net Carbs: 8g, Protein: 34g

Ingredients

Sesame mayonnaise

- Mayonnaise ¾ c

- Sesame oil 1 tsp

- Lime juice ½ tbsp

- Salt and pepper>> to taste

Beef

- Olive oil 1 tbsp

- Fish sauce 1 tbsp

- Grated fresh ginger 1 tbsp

- Chili flakes 1 tsp

- Ribeye steaks 2/3 lb.

Salad

- Cherry tomatoes 3 oz

- Cucumber 2 oz

- Lettuce 3 oz

- Red onion 1/2

- Sesame seeds 1 tsp

- Fresh cilantro

- Scallions 2

Instruction

- ❖ Through combining mayo with the lime juice and sesame oil, make the sesame mayonnaise. With pepper and salt, season. Set it aside.
- ❖ Combine all of the beef marinade components and put them in a plastic container. Add the beef then marinate it at room temp for 15 mins or more.

- ❖ Divide all of the chopped vegetables into two bowls, except the scallions.
- ❖ Over med heat, heat a med frying pan. In a dry skillet, add the sesame seeds and toast for a few minutes or till lightly browned & fragrant. Set it aside.
- ❖ On all sides with the paper towels, pat dry the meat. Sear on each side for a min or two at high heat, then decrease heat to med-low, cook till beef is med, and then to the cutting board move.
- ❖ Fry the scallions in the same pan for a minute.
- ❖ Cut the beef into thin strips across the grain. Place on top of vegetables the scallions and beef.
- ❖ Serve with sesame mayonnaise a dollop on the hand and finish with the roasted sesame seeds.

Venezuelan Keto Chicken Salad

(Ready in about 20 mins | Serving 4| Difficulty: Easy)

Per serving: Kcal: 384, Fat: 30g, Net Carbs: 1g, Protein: 25g

Ingredients

- Chicken breasts 1 lb.

- Salt 1 tsp

- Olive oil 2 tbsp

- Water 1 c

- mayonnaise 2 tbsp

- ripe avocado, chopped 1

- Minced fresh cilantro ¼ c

Instructions

❖ All over the chicken breast.

❖ Heat a large skillet with half of the olive oil over medium heat. When it comes to temperature, add breast to chicken and sear on each side for 4 minutes. Pour the water to the skillet & put a tight-fitting lid on it. Let it cook for 3-5 mins or until the water cooks off.

❖ Remove the chicken and shred it from the skillet. Let the salad cool down before making it.

❖ For the salad, in a large bowl, mix all the ingredients until well combined & creamy.

❖ Taste & adjust salt as needed.

Avocado Egg Salad

(Ready in about 15 mins | Serving 4| Difficulty: Easy)

Per serving: Kcal: 269, Fat: 21g, Carbs: 8g, Protein: 11g

Ingredients

- Hard-boiled eggs, diced 4
- Avocado, diced 1
- Green onions, sliced 2
- Low-sodium bacon crumbled 4 slices
- Nonfat plain yogurt ¼ c
- Low-fat sour cream 1 tbsp
- Lime, juiced 1
- Snipped fresh dill 1 tbsp
- Salt ¼ tsp
- Fresh ground pepper 1/8 tsp
- Dill & crumbled bacon, for garnishing

Instructions

- ❖ Put each egg in the cavity of a muffin tin & hard "boil" in the oven at 325F for 30 minutes.
- ❖ Remove eggs from the oven and then transfer them to ice water; peel & dice.
- ❖ Combine the diced eggs, avocado, green onions, & bacon in a salad bowl; set aside.
- ❖ Whisk yogurt, sour cream, lime juice, dill, salt, & pepper together in a mixing bowl; whisk until well blended.
- ❖ Add the egg salad with yogurt mixture; mix until combined.
- ❖ Garnish with crumbled bacon and dill.
- ❖ Serve.
- ❖ You can also spread the salad over 4 slices of bread; add the tomatoes & lettuce to make a delicious sandwich of egg salad.
- ❖ Keep refrigerated.

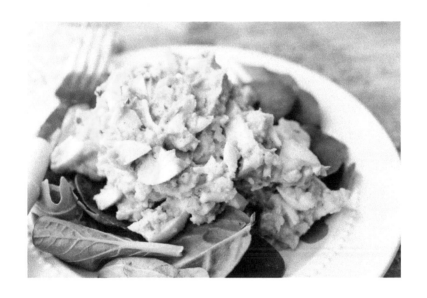

Keto Low-Carb Strawberry Jello Salad

(Ready in about 10 mins | Serving 10| Difficulty: Easy)

Per serving: Cal: 255, Fat: 23g, Net Carbs: 4g, Protein: 4g

Ingredients

- Heavy whipping cream 1 c

- Vanilla extract, unsweetened ½ tsp

- Mascarpone cheese softened 8 oz

- 4% fat large curd cottage cheese 1 c

- 1 box sugar-free strawberry jello (6 oz)

- Chopped walnuts ¼ c

- Unsweetened shredded coconut 1/3 c

- Chopped strawberries 2 cups

Instructions

- ❖ Beat the heavy whipping cream & vanilla in a medium bowl until stiff peaks form.
- ❖ Fold in the mascarpone cheese carefully until fully incorporated.
- ❖ Gently stir in jello-free cottage cheese & powdered sugar, then mix well.
- ❖ Fold in walnuts, coconut & strawberries.
- ❖ If desired, spoon into a mold & chill for 4 hours before serving.
- ❖ Dip the container in hot water for about twenty seconds (longer if necessary) to unmold, and then flip over to a serving platter.
- ❖ If desired, garnish with additional strawberries (not listed in nutrition info).
- ❖ Store leftovers in the refrigerator in an airtight container for up to 5 days. Do not freeze.

Blue Cheese Coleslaw

(Ready in about 10 mins | Serving 4| Difficulty: Easy)

Per serving: kcal: 129, Fat: 8g, Carbs: 13g, Protein: 3g

Ingredients

- Original cheese dressing blue 6 tbsp

- Buttermilk 2 tbsp

- Chopped Green cabbage ½

- Chopped Red cabbage 1/2

- Thickly sliced green onion ½ c

- Celery seed 2 tsp

- Salt & ground black pepper

- Crumbled blue cheese 1/4

Instructions

- ❖ Mix the cheese dressing (blue) & buttermilk until the thickness is the one you prefer.

- ❖ Slice thickly, the green onions until around 1/2 c of green onion have been sliced.
- ❖ Use a Mandoline Slicer or a long knife to cut the entire cabbage in thin strips; now chop the cabbage strips coarsely.
- ❖ In a large bowl, mix the diced green cabbage, red cabbage chopped, and green onion sliced, then stir in the dressing desired amount.
- ❖ Add the seed of celery, blue cheese crumbled (if used), and salt & pepper fresh ground to taste & stir a few times gently.
- ❖ Serve immediately.
- ❖ If this recipe is more than you're going to eat at one time,
- ❖ Store the dressing mixture and the mixture of cabbage / green onion separately in the fridge & combine and season the salad just before eating the leftovers.

Keto Asian Noodles Salad with Peanut Sauce

(Ready in about 10 mins | Serving 4| Difficulty: Easy)

Per serving: Cal: 212, Fat: 16g, Net Carbs: 6g, Protein: 7g

Ingredients

For the salad:

- Shredded red cabbage 1 c

- Shredded green cabbage 1 c

- Chopped scallions ¼ c

- Chopped cilantro ¼ c

- Shirataki noodles 4 c

- Chopped peanuts ¼ c

For the dressing:

- Minced ginger 2 tbsp

- Minced Garlic 1 tsp

33

- Filtered water ½ c

- Lime juice 1 tbsp

- Toasted sesame oil 1 tbsp

- Wheat-free soy sauce 1 tbsp

- Fish sauce 1 tbsp

- Sugar-free peanut butter ¼ c

- Cayenne pepper ¼ tsp

- Kosher salt ½ tsp

- Granulated erythritol sweetener 1 tbsp

Instructions

- ❖ Combine all the ingredients for the salad in a large bowl.
- ❖ Combine all the ingredients for the dressing in a blender or magic bullet.
- ❖ Mix until smooth.
- ❖ Pour the salad over the dressing & toss to coat.
- ❖ Serve immediately, or store in the refrigerator in an airtight container for up to 5 days. Do not freeze

BLT Lobster Rolls Salad – Low-Carb and Paleo

(Ready in about 10 mins | Serving 4| Difficulty: Easy)

Per serving: Cal: 330, Fat: 28g, Net Carbs: 3g, Protein: 19g

Ingredients

For the lobster salad:

- Cooked lobster meat, chopped 2 c

- Cauliflower floret, cooked until tender 1&1/2 c

- Sugar-free mayonnaise ½ c

- Tarragon leaves chopped 1 tsp

To serve:

- Romaine lettuce leaves 8

- Chopped tomatoes ½ c

- Cooked bacon, chopped ½ c

Instructions

For the salad:

❖ Combine the cooked lobster in a medium bowl with cooked cauliflower, mayonnaise, and tarragon. Stir until creamy and well combined.

To serve:

❖ Put the leaves of lettuce on a platter. Divide the mixture of the lobster salad into the 8 leaves. Sprinkle with bacon & chopped tomatoes.

❖ Serve at room temperature or cold.

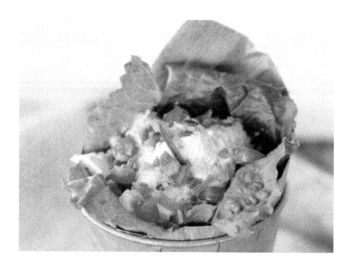

Rosemary Avocado, Chicken & Bacon Salad

(Ready in about 35 mins | Serving 2| Difficulty: Easy)

Per serving: Cal: 324.2, Fat: 28.2g, carbs: 8.6g, Protein: 10.7g

Ingredients

- Thick-cut bacon 4 slices

- Boneless, chicken breasts ½ lb.

- Salt and pepper >> to taste

- Olive oil 1 tbsp

- Minced fresh rosemary 2 tbsp

- Spring greens and/or butter lettuce 6 c

- Watercress 1 bunch

- Cherry tomatoes halved 1 c

- Avocado, thinly sliced 1

Rosemary vinaigrette

- Dijon mustard 2 tsp

- Olive oil ¼ c

- Red wine vinegar ¼ c

- Minced fresh rosemary 1 tsp

- Salt and pepper>> to taste

Instructions

- ❖ Heat a large skillet and add the bacon over medium-low heat. Cook until crispy and render the fat. Place the bacon on a paper towel to drain any remaining grease.
- ❖ The chicken is seasoned with salt & pepper. Cover with the rosemary. In the same skillet, add the chicken over med-high heat, & cook on both sides, about 5 to 6 minutes each side, until golden and crisp. Remove the chicken and let it sit for a moment while the salad is being assembled, then slice.

❖ Toss the greens along with the watercress & the tomatoes. Use the sliced chicken, bacon & avocado to top. Drizzle your vinaigrette with the rosemary.

Rosemary vinaigrette

❖ Whisk mustard, olive oil & vinegar together. Whisk in the rosemary & sprinkle with salt and pepper.

Low-Carb Broccoli Salad

Ready in about 10 mins | Serving 8| Difficulty: Easy)

Per serving: Kcal: 287, Fat: 26.7g, Net Carbs: 2.7g, Protein: 5.94g

Ingredients

- Broccoli 6 c
- Chopped Onion 1/3
- Mayonnaise 1 c
- Chopped Almonds ½ c
- Red vinegar 2 tbsp
- Chopped cooked bacon 8 slices
- Salt & pepper

Instructions

- ❖ Combine broccoli, bacon, onion & almonds in a large bowl.
- ❖ Mix mayonnaise, vinegar, salt & pepper in a separate bowl, then in a small bowl.
- ❖ Pour broccoli mixture over the dressing and stir until the coat becomes even.
- ❖ Cover and chill for at least an hour, until it's ready to serve.

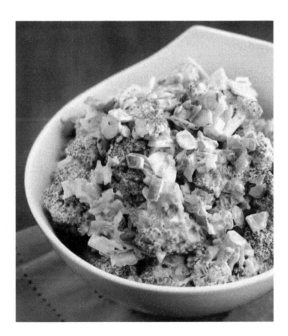

Chicken Fajita Wedge Salad

(Ready in about 10 mins | Serving 4 | Difficulty: Medium)

Per serving: Cal: 271, Fat: 17g, Carbs: 18g, Protein: 12g

Ingredients

- Boneless skinless chicken breasts 2
- Chili powder ¾ tsp
- Cumin ¼ tsp
- Creole seasoning ½ tsp
- Head iceberg lettuce 1/2
- Chopped tomato 1
- Finely diced red onion 1/4
- Diced green bell pepper 1/4c
- Diced cucumber1/2 c
- Shredded cheddar cheese ½ c
- Salsa 3 tbsp
- Ranch dressing ¼ c

- Diced avocado 1
- Cilantro 1 tbsp

Instructions

- ❖ Season the chicken breasts with chili powder, cumin, and Creole seasoning on both sides.
- ❖ Grill for about 18 minutes over medium heat or until chicken is cooked through. Remove from heat & allow a few minutes to rest.
- ❖ Again, cut the 1/2 head of lettuce into half. Put each of the wedges on a plate. Top with bell peppers, tomatoes, onion, cucumber & shredded cheese.
- ❖ Combine salsa & ranch dressing. Drizzle each wedge over. Garnish with Cilantro and Avocado.
- ❖ Slice the chicken alongside the wedge & serve it.

Muffaletta Salad

(Ready in about 15 mins | Serving 4 | Difficulty: Medium)

Per serving: Cal: 2850, Fat: 252g, Carbs: 43g, Protein: 111g

Ingredients

- 1 bag Romaine lettuce 9 oz

- Celery stalk, chopped 1

- Red bell pepper 1

- Red onion, finely chopped 1/2

- Sliced salami, chopped 4 oz

- Sliced soppressata, chopped 4 oz

- Sliced mortadella, chopped 4 oz

- Sliced Provolone cheese, chopped 4 oz

- 1 jar giardiniera salad, drained & chopped 16 oz

- Chopped kalamata olives ½ c

- Pepperoncini, finely chopped 6-8

- Shredded Parmesan cheese 2 tbsp

Dressing

- Red wine vinegar 3 tbsp

- Olive oil or vegetable oil ¼ c

- Cloves garlic, finely minced 1

- Dried oregano 1/4

- Dried basil 1/4

- Salt and pepper>> to taste

Instructions

- ❖ Combine all the ingredients for the salad in a large bowl.
- ❖ Whisk all the dressing ingredients together and season with salt and pepper to taste.
- ❖ Toss on salad dressing.

Salmon & Avocado Caesar Salad

Ready in about 10 mins | Serving 2| Difficulty: Easy)

Per serving: Kcal: 828, Fat: 58.2g, Carbs: 13.5g, Protein: 49.5g

Ingredients

Salad:

- Cubed ciabatta/sourdough ½ c

- 5oz salmon fillets fresh, skin off 5 oz

- Garlic powder 1 tsp

- Pinch Salt

- Diced bacon ¼ c

- Juice of 1/2 lemon

- Eggs, boiled 2

- Lettuce 2 c

- Avocado, sliced 1

- Parmesan cheese ½ c

Dressing:

- Egg mayo 2 tbsp

- Greek yogurt/sour cream 3 tbsp

- Olive oil one tbsp

- Crushed clove garlic 1

- Finely chopped Anchovy fillet 1

- Lemon juice 1 tbsp

- Parmesan grated cheese 1 tbsp

- Salt & pepper

Instructions

- ❖ The oven is preheated to med-high heat to grill/broil settings. Place cubed bread on the oven tray; then drizzle it with olive oil & bake until crispy in oven (on the middle shelf).
- ❖ Rub garlic powder & salt to the salmon fillets.

- ❖ Heat a pan/skillet (non-stick) with olive oil drizzle & fry salmon until both sides are golden and cooked according to as you like.
- ❖ The salmon is removed; squeeze the juice of a lemon over each filet and set it aside on the warm plate. Put the bacon in the same saucepan and fry until golden & crispy.
- ❖ Boil/poach the eggs as you like while the bacon is frying. Put a water small pot & white vinegar 2 tsp on the boil on med heat if poaching.
- ❖ Create a quick whirlpool with a spoon in the center of water & crack the egg in the middle while that water is swirling.
- ❖ As the whites start to set, some of the water is spooned over the yolk until it starts changing color with a cloudy white top, & immediately the egg is removed with the slotted spoon.

Caesar dressing:

- ❖ In a small bowl, combine mayo, oil, garlic, yogurt, lemon juice, anchovies, & parmesan.

❖ Mix well/blend when using the blender, until it's combined; add pepper & salt to taste, and blend/mix until smooth again. Taste test.

Assemble salad:

❖ Combine the salmon & bacon with lettuce; slices of avocado; parmesan cheese shaved; & croutons. Pour the dressing; combine well; put on top the eggs, and serve.

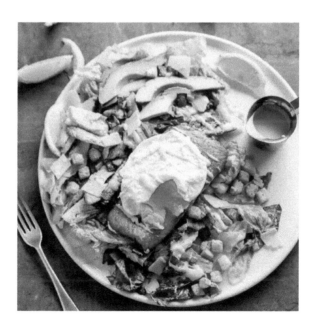

20. Cauliflower Potato Salad - Low Carb and Paleo

Ready in about 40 mins | Serving 4| Difficulty: Easy)

Per serving: Kcal: 320, Fat: 27g, Net Carbs: 5g, Protein: 5g

Ingredients

- Cauliflower 2

- Olive oil 2 tbsp

- Sea salt ½ tsp

- Black pepper ¼ tsp

- Avocado mayonnaise 1.5 c

- Yellow mustard ¼ c

- Dill pickles, diced 1 c

- White onion 1 c

- Celery, diced ½ c

- Hard-boiled eggs 6

- Apple cider vinegar 1 tbsp
- Paprika >>for topping

Instructions

❖ To 375 ° F preheat the oven. Line 2 large parchment-laden baking sheets.

❖ Dice the cauliflower into 1-inch cubes & add olive oil & salt and pepper to taste. Spread over a single layer onto the baking sheets. Bake for 30 mins, until the tops begin to turn golden. Let's just cool down.

❖ hard boil your eggs while the cauliflower bakes.

❖ Combine the remaining ingredients into a large bowl, add the cauliflower & 4 diced eggs, toss to coat.

❖ Save with salt & pepper & add more if necessary. Layer the salad in a serving dish, slice the remaining egg thinly over the top & lay them over. Sprinkle on paprika, chill until ready for serving.

Iceberg Wedge Salad

(Ready in about 15 mins | Serving 4 | Difficulty: Easy)

Per serving: Kcal: 201, Fat: 13g, Carbs: 8g, Protein: 11g

Ingredients

For the dressing-

- Plain Greek yogurt ¼ c

- Sour cream 3 tbsp

- Mayonnaise 1 tbsp

- Milk 3 tbsp

- Worcestershire>> dash

- Blue cheese crumbles ¼ c

- White balsamic vinegar 2 tsp

- Salt & pepper >>to taste

For the wedge's salads-

- One iceberg lettuce cut into four

- Bacon cooked & crumbled 1/3 c

- Hard-boiled eggs chopped 4

- Grape tomatoes sliced in half 10

- Extra blue cheese crumbled 1-2 tbsp per salad

- Chives

Instructions

- ❖ Whisk all ingredients together in a small bowl to dress. Put on aside.
- ❖ Place wedges of iceberg lettuce on two diner plates cut side up. Gentle Drizzle with dressing. Top with bacon, eggs, tomatoes, chives, and extra blue cheese. Serve

Cobb Coastal Salad with Cilantro Lemon Dressing

(Ready in about 10 mins | Serving 3 | Difficulty: Easy)

Per serving: Kcal: 333, Fat: 21.7g, Carbs: 8.9g, Protein: 27.2g

Ingredients

Cream cilantro lemon dressing

- Paleo mayonnaise ¼ c

- Minced cilantro 3 tbsp

- Water 1 tbsp

- Fresh lemon juice 2 tsp

- Zest of lemon 1

- Garlic powder ¼ tsp

- Sea salt ½ tsp

Coastal cobb salad

- Chopped romaine lettuce 6 c

- Cooked shrimp 6 oz

- Cooked chicken breast, sliced 4 oz

- Boiled eggs, halved 2

- Crumbled cooked bacon

- Avocado, chopped

- Grape or cherry tomatoes halved 1 c

- Chopped cilantro ½ c

- Green onion sliced 1

Instructions

Cilantro Creamy lemon dressing

- ❖ Mix the ingredients by an immersion blender or hand or the food processor to blend them.
- ❖ Store in the fridge until necessary.

Coastal cobb salad

❖ Put salad together on a large platter. Line the romaine lettuce platter and then arrange the toppings.

❖ Serve with creamy lemon cilantro dressing.

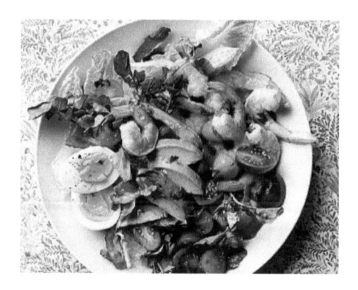

Creamy Low-Carb Shrimp & Cauliflower Salad

(Ready in about 15 mins | Serving 8 | Difficulty: Easy)

Per serving: Cal: 182, Fat: 14g, Net Carbs: 2g, Protein: 13g

Ingredients

For the salad:

- Cauliflower florets 5 c

- Cooked large shrimp chilled and cut lengthwise in half 2 c

- Diced celery 1/3 c

- Sliced canned black olives ½ c

- Fresh dill, chopped 1 tbsp

For the dressing:

- Mayonnaise ½ c

- Celery seed ¼ tsp

- Lemon juice 2 tbsp

- Granulated sugar substitute 2 tsp

- Apple cider vinegar 1 tsp

- Kosher salt ¼ tsp

- Ground black pepper 1/8 tsp

Instructions

- ❖ In a large bowl, combine the salad ingredients, and toss gently.
- ❖ Combine the ingredients for the dressing in a small bowl & whisk together until smooth.
- ❖ Pour the dressing & stir gently until well covered.
- ❖ If possible, chill up for half an hour to let the flavors meld.
- ❖ Serve cold.

Keto Broccoli Slaw – Low-Carb & Gluten-Free

(Ready in about 35 mins | Serving 6 | Difficulty: Easy)

Per serving: kcal: 110, Fat: 10g, Net Carbs: 2g, Protein: 2g

Ingredients

- Olive oil 1 tbsp

- Sugar-free mayonnaise 1/3 c

- Apple cider vinegar 1&1/2 tbsp

- Dijon mustard 1 tbsp

- Granulated sugar substitute 2 tbsp

- Celery seeds 1 tsp

- Kosher salt ½ tsp

- Black pepper ¼ tsp

- Bagged broccoli slaw 4 c

Instructions

- ❖ Whisk together the olive oil, mayonnaise, apple cider vinegar, mustard, sugar substitute, celery seeds, salt, & pepper in a large bowl until completely combined.
- ❖ Add the slaw on broccoli. Toss to coat. Serve chilled

Salad Green Bean

(Ready in about 27 mins | Serving 6 | Difficulty: Easy)

Per serving: Cal: 232, Fat: 20g, Carbs: 13g, Protein: 5g

Ingredients:

- Green beans fresh 1 lb.

- Sliced palm hearts 2 cups

- Kalamata olives/black olives 3/4 cup, sliced in half and drained

- Bell pepper red diced roasted 1 cup

- Feta cheese crumbled 1/2 cup

- Black pepper fresh ground

Dressing ingredients:

- Balsamic vinegar 1 T

- lemon juice fresh-squeezed 2 T

- Olive oil 1/3 cup

- Lemon zest 1 tsp.

- Fresh oregano chopped 2 T

- Fresh basil chopped 2 T

Instructions

- ❖ Trim green beans end.
- ❖ Cut the beans into about 2" long pieces.
- ❖ Steam beans in a big pot having a lid tight-fitting or a vegetable steamer (electric), using a steamer insert until they are some tender-crisp.
- ❖ When beans are tender as you would like them, take off the steamer and immediately plunge into an ice water bowl to halt the cooking.
- ❖ Remove the beans to a colander and allow them to drain and cool for about 15 mins, then spread the beans on towels on paper and then blot dry.
- ❖ While the beans cook, slice and drain the palm hearts, drain & red peppers chop, drain and cut olives in half, then measure the feta.
- ❖ Combine lemon juice, balsamic vinegar, olive oil, chopped oregano, lemon zest & chopped basil &

process until the herbs are chopped very thinly, and the dressing is well mixed.

- ❖ Combine drained beans and sliced palm heart, olive halves, & red pepper chopped to assemble the salad.
- ❖ To moisten salad, add dressing as required and gently combine.
- ❖ Add the feta cheese & stir to make the feta barely mix.
- ❖ Grind black pepper & serve straight away.
- ❖ This can keep inside the refrigerator for several days but bring the leftovers to room temp before serving.

Anti-Pasta Cauliflower Salad – Low-Carb & Gluten-Free

(Ready in about 75 mins | Serving 8 | Difficulty: Easy)

Per serving: Cal: 102, Fat: 8g, Carbs: 4g, Protein: 3g

Ingredients

- Chopped Raw cauliflower 2 c

- Chopped Radicchio ½ c

- Chopped Artichoke hearts ½ c

- Chopped fresh basil 1/3 c

- Grated parmesan ½ c

- Chopped Sundried tomatoes 3 tbsp

- Chopped Kalamata olives 3 tbsp

- Minced Clove Garlic1

- Balsamic vinegar 3 tbsp

- Olive oil 3 tbsp

- Salt & pepper

Instructions

❖ First, cook five minutes in the microwave the chopped cauliflower. Do not add any seasoning or liquid to it. Simply spread and zap it on the safe microwave platter. Let cool down the cauliflower while the further ingredients are prepared.

❖ In a medium bowl, combine the artichoke heart, radicchio, basil, parmesan, olives, sundried tomatoes, & garlic.

❖ Whisk the vinegar and olive oil together in a smaller bowl, then pour over salad. Toss it to coat, and sprinkle with salt & pepper. Can be chilled or served at room temperature

Bacon & Eggs Spinach Salad

(Ready in about 30 mins | Serving 10 | Difficulty: Easy)

Per serving: Cal: 248, Fat: 20g, Carbs: 5.3g, Protein: 12g

Ingredients

- Clove garlic 1
- Kosher salt ½ tsp
- Red wine vinegar 2 tbsp
- Dijon 1 tbsp
- Olive oil 3 tbsp
- Freshly ground pepper >>to taste
- Spinach leaves 12 c
- Hard-boiled eggs peeled & chopped 4
- Bacon, cooked & crumbled 4 slices

Instructions

❖ Smash the garlic clove and peel it. Mince with the side of a chef's knife and mash with salt to form a paste. Scrap into a medium-sized bowl. Whisk in Dijon and Vinegar. In oil, whisk gradually. Season with pepper.

❖ Place a large salad bowl with spinach, eggs, and bacon. Pour over the salad dressing & then toss to combine.

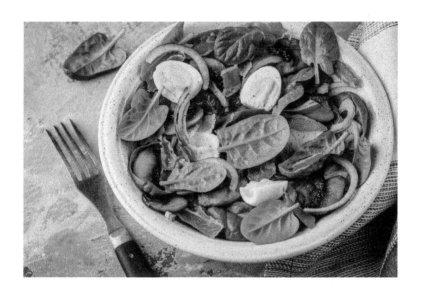

Buffalo Chicken Chopped Salad

(Ready in about 35 mins | Serving 6-8 | Difficulty: Easy)

Per serving: Cal: 642, Fat: 46.4g, Net carbs: 8.7g, Protein: 42.2g

Chicken Ingredients

- Chicken breasts boneless 2

- Buffalo sauce ½ c

Salad

- Lettuce Head chopped 1

- Carrots shredded 1 c

- Celery Chopped 1 c

- Chopped Cucumber 1

- Diced Avocado1

- Diced Tomatoes 1 c

- Crumbled Blue cheese ½ c

Dressing

- Ranch dressing one c
- Cheese crumbles Blue ¼ c
- Sauce Buffalo wing ¼ c

Instructions

- ❖ Add chicken & buffalo sauce into a small bowl. Mix until the chicken is covered with sauce.
- ❖ Add the lettuce, celery, cucumber, carrots, avocado & tomatoes into a large bowl. Mix.
- ❖ In individual bowls, add a salad. Top with about ½ cup of chicken buffalo and crumbles of blue cheese, each salad.
- ❖ In a small bowl or jar, combine the ranch dressing, buffalo sauce, and blue cheese dressing. Serve to dress on the side & add to each salad bowl a few tbsp of homemade ranch dressing spicy.
- ❖ Enjoy it.

Low-Carb - Chinese Chicken Salad

(Ready in about 30 mins | Serving 8 | Difficulty: Easy)

Per serving: Cal: 263, Fat: 16g, Net Carbs: 3g, Protein: 24g

Ingredients

For the chicken:

- Boneless, chicken thigh 1.5 lb.

- Water 4 c

- Garlic powder ½ tsp

- Onion powder ½ tsp

- Kosher salt 1 tsp

- Gluten-free soy sauce ¼ c

- Minced ginger 1 tbsp

For the salad:

- Shredded white cabbage 2 c

- Shredded savoy or Napa cabbage 2 c

- Sliced baby cucumbers 2 c

- Sliced scallions ½ c

- Radishes cut into matchsticks ½ c

- Cilantro, chopped ¼ c

- Sesame seeds 2 tbsp

For the dressing:

- Gluten-free soy sauce ¼ c

- Sesame oil 1 tsp

- Unsweetened rice wine vinegar 1/3 c

- Granulated sugar substitute 1 tbsp

- Avocado oil 3 tbsp

- Hot Chinese mustard ¼ tsp

- Unsweetened ginger paste 1 tbsp

Instructions

To make the chicken:

- ❖ Combine all the ingredients and bring to a boil in a large saucepan.
- ❖ Turn the heat down and cook the chicken for 15-20 mins, or until cooked. Remove the chicken & allow it to cook for a couple of minutes.
- ❖ Shred with two forks or cut with a knife, making sure that any ligaments are removed, etc.

To make the salad:

- ❖ Combine the cabbages, then spread them over a platter or bowl.
- ❖ Arrange the cukes around the bowl or platter outside and leave room in the center for the chicken.
- ❖ Sprinkle on the cilantro, radish matchsticks, and scallions. Then pile the chicken in the platter or bowl center. Sprinkle with sesame seeds.

To make the dressing:

❖ Combine all the dressing components in a magic bullet or blender & blend until smooth and complete.

❖ Taste the seasoning to check & then pour over the salad several minutes before serving.

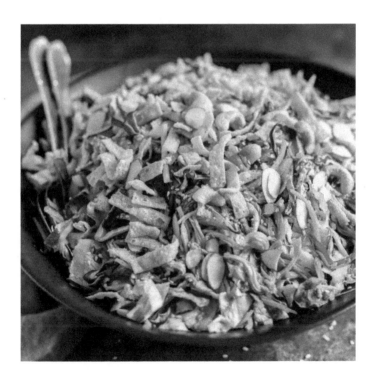

Creamy dilled cucumber salad

(Ready in about 10 mins | Serving 4| Difficulty: Easy)

Per serving: Cal: 47, Fat: 1g, Carbs: 8g, Protein: 2g

Ingredients

- Large cucumbers, sliced 2
- Red onion, sliced ¼ c
- Greek yogurt ¼ c
- Lemon, juice & zest 1
- Dill, chopped 2 tbsp
- Salt and pepper >>to taste
- Clove garlic, grated 1

Directions

- ❖ Mix it all up & enjoy it.
- ❖ Option: Chill the salad in the refrigerator for 30 minutes to allow the flavors to mingle.
- ❖ Option: Add some teaspoon of sugar or honey for a touch of sweetness.

74

Pastrami Salad with Fried Egg & Croutons - Keto

Ready in about 20 mins | Serving 2| Difficulty: Easy)

Per serving: Kcal: 696, Fat: 57g, Net Carbs: 5g, Protein: 38g

Ingredients

- Mayonnaise ½ c

- Dijon mustard 2 tbsp

- Shallot 1

- Dill pickle 1

- Lettuce 4 oz

- Pastrami 8 oz

- eggs 4

- low-carb parmesan croutons 4

Instructions

- ❖ Start making the parmesan croutons low carb, if you don't already have them on hand.
- ❖ Mix mayonnaise & mustard & set aside.
- ❖ Put the lettuce on 2 slabs. Cut the onion & put it on top.
- ❖ Lengthwise cut the pickled cucumber into four pieces and place it on the lettuce.
- ❖ Add pastrami & a generous amount of mayonnaise on the mustard.
- ❖ The eggs should be fried just before serving the salad. Sunnyside faces up or over and serves with parmesan croutons immediately.

Keto Avocado, Bacon & Goat-Cheese Salad

(Ready in about 30 mins | Serving 4| Difficulty: Easy)

Per serving: Kcal: 1251, Fat: 123g, Net Carbs: 6g, Protein: 27g

Ingredients

- Goat cheese 8 oz

- Bacon 8 oz

- Avocados 2

- Arugula lettuce 4 oz

- Walnuts 4 oz

Dressing

- Lemon juice 1 tbsp

- mayonnaise ½ c

- Olive oil ½ c

- Heavy whipping cream 2 tbsp

- Salt and pepper>> to taste

Instructions

- ❖ Preheat the oven to 200 ° C and place the parchment paper in a baking platter.
- ❖ Sliced the goat cheese into slices of round half-inch (~1 cm) & place them in the baking platter. Bake until golden on the upper rack.
- ❖ Fry the bacon in a saucepan until it is crispy.
- ❖ Cut the avocado into pieces & put the arugula on top. Add the goat cheese and fried bacon. Sprinkle nuts on top.
- ❖ Make the dressing with the lime juice, mayonnaise, olive oil & cream, using an immersion blender. To taste, season with salt & pepper.

Cajun Keto Chicken Salad with Guacamole

(Ready in about 35 mins | Serving 2| Difficulty: Easy)

Per serving: Kcal: 927, Fat: 65g, Net Carbs: 20g, Protein: 57g

Ingredients

Cajun spice mix

- Sweet paprika powder 4 tsp

- Dried thyme 3 tbsp

- Garlic cloves, minced 2

- Pinch of cayenne pepper

- Olive oil 1 tbsp

- Boneless, chicken breasts 1 lb.

- Sugar snap peas 7 oz

- Tomatoes 4

- Olive oil 3 tbsp

- Salt & ground black pepper>> to taste

- Avocado 1

- Juice of 1 lemon

- Arugula lettuce 2 oz

Instructions

- ❖ Make the Cajun spice mix in a bowl. Combine the olive oil, the paprika, thyme, garlic, cayenne. Cut into long strips of chicken. Add the chicken & coat with a mixture of spices. May marinate the chicken for at least 5 mins.
- ❖ Bring water to a boil with a saucepan. Add the peas & continue cooking until al dente. Drain well.
- ❖ The tomatoes are quarter, core, & seed. Cut the tomatoes into small wedges. Do this over a sieve & keep the juices for the vinaigrette.

- ❖ Make a tomato juice vinaigrette with 2/3 of the olive oil, salt & pepper.
- ❖ Cut the avocado, pit, and peel; put the flesh in a bowl & add the lemon juice. Sprinkle with salt & pepper, & mash.
- ❖ In a skillet over moderate heat, cook the chicken in the rest of the olive oil for 10 to 15 mins, until cooked through.
- ❖ Toss the tomatoes & peas with the arugula & arrange them on plates.
- ❖ Divide the guacamole & chicken strips between the plates. Serve the vinaigrette separately.

Keto Kohl Slaw

(Ready in about 15 mins | Serving 4| Difficulty: Easy

Per serving: Kcal: 405, Fat: 41g, Net Carbs: 3g, Protein: 2g

Ingredients

- Kohlrabis 1 lb.

- mayonnaise or vegan mayonnaise 1 c

- Salt & pepper>> to taste

- Fresh parsley

Instructions

❖ Peel Kohlrabi. Be sure to cut any hard, woody parts away. Shave, slice, and/or finely shred it and place it in a bowl.

❖ Add the mayonnaise & fresh herbs as an option. Salt and pepper to taste.

Keto Cheeseburger Salad

(Ready in about 35 mins | Serving 4| Difficulty: Medium)

Per serving: Kcal: 1083, Fat: 94g, Net Carbs: 8g, Protein: 49g

Ingredients

- Seasoned ground beef

- Ground beef or ground turkey 24 oz

- Butter 4 tbsp

- Garlic powder 2 tsp

- Salt 1.5 tsp

- Ground black pepper ¼ tsp

- Toasted sesame seeds, to serve

Dressing

- Mayonnaise 1 c

- Tomato paste 1 tbsp

- Pickles, chopped 3 oz

- Yellow or Dijon mustard ½ tbsp

- White wine vinegar 1 tsp

- Salt & ground black pepper>> to taste

Salad

- Lettuce, cut into smaller lettuce leaves 4 oz

- Red onions, sliced 2 oz

- Tomatoes, sliced 9 oz

- Pickles, each cut in half widthwise 2

- Cheddar cheese, shredded 8 oz

Instructions

Seasoned ground beef

- ❖ Melt the butter in a large skillet over medium heat.

- ❖ Add beef, salt, black pepper & garlic powder to the saucepan. Mix the beef and the seasonings with a spatula and crumble, frying until browned & cooked about 15 minutes.

Dressing

- ❖ Combine all the dressing ingredients in a small bowl, then set aside.

Salad

- ❖ Organize each serving by layering every serving dish: start with lettuce, add tomatoes, beef top, cheese, red onion & pickles. In the end, drizzle the dressing on top.

PORK

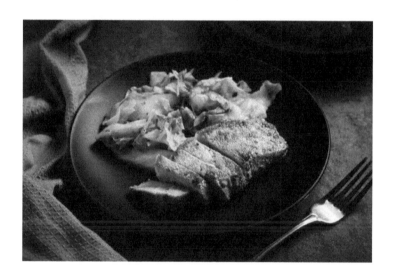

Keto Pork Burgers

(Ready in about 20 mins | Serving 4 | Difficulty: Easy)

Per serving: Cal: 601, Fat: 53g, Net Carbs: 3g, Protein: 29g

Ingredients

Ingredients list for the burger:

- Ground pork ½ lb.
- Ground beef ½ lb.
- Chili powder 1 tsp
- Onion powder 1 tbsp
- Garlic powder 1 tbsp
- Italian seasoning 1 tbsp
- Whisked egg 1
- Mustard 1 tsp
- Salt ½ tsp
- Pinch of pepper

Ingredients list for Spicy Mayo:

- Mayo ¼ c
- Hot sauce 1 tsp
- Mustard 1 tsp
- Pinch of salt

Toppings Ingredients:

- Slices of cooked bacon 8 slices
- Avocado slices or guacamole
- Fresh chopped parsley

Instructions

- ❖ Put all ingredients of the burger in a bowl and mix well. Using your hands, create tiny patties (shapes approx. 8) from the meat mixture.
- ❖ Place the patties over medium heat on a hot grill or pan, and grill for around five mins. Turn the patties carefully over and grill for

another 3 to 5 minutes, until cooked to your taste.

❖ Prepare the hot mayo by adding with the Mayo ingredients.

❖ Stack the patties with mayo & bacon.

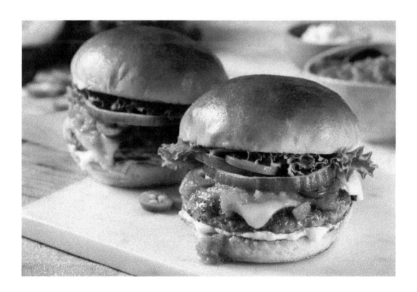

Keto Meatballs & Bok Choy

(Ready in about 45 mins | Serving 4 | Difficulty: Easy)

Per serving: Cal: 369, Fat: 21g, Net Carbs: 5g, Protein: 40g

Ingredients

Ingredients list for meatballs:

- Diced spring onion 1
- Minced garlic clove 1
- Ground pork or any other mincemeat of your choice 1.5 lb.
- Salt & pepper>> to taste
- Whisked egg 1
- Finely chopped 2 slices of bacon

Ingredients list for Bok Choy:

- Diced tomatoes ½ c
- Roughly chopped bunches of bok choy 2
- Minced garlic cloves 2

- Diced onion 1/4

- Salt & pepper>> to taste

- Avocado oil 2 tbsp

Instructions

- ❖ In a big mixing bowl, bring all the meatball's ingredients together and combine them. Using a spoon to mold meatballs like ping-pong balls.

- ❖ To 350 F, preheat the oven. Line a parchment paper baking tray and put the meatballs on the tray. Bake for 20-25 mins until the meatballs hit 140 F in internal temp.

- ❖ Apply the avocado oil to the frying pan and cook the meatballs gently, including the onions. Add the remaining ingredients and boil for 10 mins until the vegetables are soft.

Keto Meatballs with the Marinara Sauce

(Ready in about 20 mins | Serving 4 | Difficulty: Easy)

Per serving: Cal: 287, Fat: 18g, Net Carbs: 6g, Protein: 26g

Ingredients

Ingredients list for meatballs:

- Avocado oil 2 tbsp
- Ground pork 1 lb.
- Chopped parsley ¼ cup
- Whisked egg 1
- Garlic powder ½ tsp
- Salt & pepper

Ingredients list for Marinara Sauce:

- Olive oil 1 tbsp
- Chopped onion ¼ c
- Minced garlic cloves 2

- Crushed tomatoes 1 c

- Chicken broth 1 c

- Italian seasoning 1 tsp

- Lemon zest ½ tsp

- Coconut cream 2 tbsp

Instructions

Instructions for Producing Meatballs:

- ❖ In a bowl, add all the meatball components (except avocado oil).
- ❖ From the mixture, make tiny balls (you can create around 15 meatballs).
- ❖ In a sauté pan, heat the avocado oil & prepare the meatballs in tiny quantities. Flip them over before they become golden-brown.

Instructions on how to make the marinara sauce:

- ❖ Apply the olive oil, onion, and garlic in a separate saucepan and simmer until the onions become translucent but not browned.

- ❖ Add the onions, chicken broth, & Italian seasoning & bring for around ten minutes to a gentle boil.
- ❖ Apply the lemon zest & cream and allow to cook for another ten min. Serve with cauliflower rice or veggies.

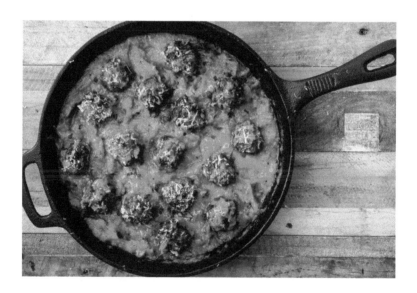

Keto Italian Dairy-Free Eggplant Pork Rollatinis

(Ready in about 30 mins | Serving 6 | Difficulty: Easy)

Per serving: Cal: 157, Fat: 4g, Net Carbs: 13g, Protein: 19g

Ingredients

- Ground pork 1 lb.
- Eggplants 2
- Egg 1
- Onion powder 1 tbsp
- Garlic powder 1 tsp
- Italian seasoning 1 tbsp
- Can of tomato sauce or marinara sauce 400 g
- Salt & pepper>> to taste

Instructions

- ❖ To 400 F, preheat the oven.
- ❖ Cut the eggplant into small, long strips. Salt well, then push the paper towels to drain extra. Leave in for ten mins.
- ❖ Meanwhile, mix the spices in a little bowl (garlic powder, Italian seasoning, onion powder, salt & pepper).
- ❖ Merge the egg & ground pork in another dish and 1/2 seasoning.
- ❖ Mix the tomato sauce with the remaining seasoning.
- ❖ Spoon the pork mixture evenly on the eggplant's slices and roll up the slices (does around 12 rollatini).
- ❖ Place flat rolls on a baking plate. (Use a cocktail stick to protect the rolls, if necessary)
- ❖ Bake thirty mins. Using a meat thermometer to verify that the pork hits an internal temp of 145F.

- ❖ (You should scatter a little mozzarella on top of the rollatini 10 min from the end of the baking period if you like to apply cheese to the dish.)
- ❖ Heat the sauce in a pan & then pour on over rollatini.

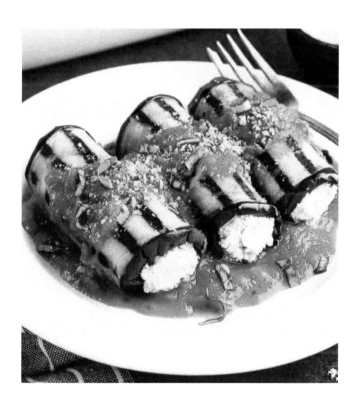

Keto Spicy Pork Meatballs

(Ready in about 20 mins | Serving 4 | Difficulty: Easy)

Per serving: Cal: 369, Fat: 27g, Net Carbs: 6g, Protein: 26g

Ingredients

For the meatballs –

- ground pork 1lb.
- whisked egg 1
- minced garlic cloves 4
- basil leaves 2 tbsp
- Hot sauce 2 tsp
- chili flakes 1 tsp
- Salt & pepper>> to taste
- Olive oil ¼ c

For the sauce –

- Olive oil 2 tbsp
- Diced onion 1/4

- Tomato sauce 220g

- Diced bell pepper 1

- Diced chili pepper 1

- Basil leaves 1 c

- Salt & pepper>>to taste

Instructions

- ❖ Combine all of the meatball components and shape 12 meatballs.

- ❖ In 1/4 cup olive oil, pan-fry the meatballs until golden. Then add the sauce's additional ingredients (excluding the basil leaves) & boil for 10 mins. Season to taste, with salt & pepper.

- ❖ Serve with pasta filled with zucchini or spaghetti squash.

Keto-Friendly Coffee-Flavored Pork Chops

(Ready in about 20 mins | Serving 2 | Difficulty: Easy)

Ingredients

Pork chops ingredients:

- 2 pork chops
- 2 tbsp olive oil or avocado oil, to cook with

Rub Ingredients:

- 1 tsp ground coffee
- ½ tsp ground cumin
- ½ tsp garlic powder
- ½ tsp smoked paprika
- ¼ tsp chili powder
- ¼ tsp salt
- ½ tsp black pepper

Garnish:

- 1 tbsp chopped parsley

Instructions

- ❖ Prepare your seasoning by mixing all the rub ingredients in a bowl.

- ❖ Wash and pat dry the pork chops. Rub them on each side with the mixture. Make sure you cover them completely.

- ❖ If you have time, place the pork chops in the refrigerator overnight.

- ❖ Take the pork chops out of the fridge and let them come to room temperature (approximately 30 minutes). Meanwhile, preheat the oven to 350 F (175 C).

- ❖ Add the cooking oil to a skillet and heat to high heat. Add the pork chops and cook them for 2-3 minutes on each side.

- ❖ Place the pan in the oven (or place the chops onto a baking pan) and let the pork chops cook for another 10 minutes in the oven.

- ❖ Let the meat rest for at least 10 minutes before enjoying.

Super Easy Pork Chops

(Ready in about 30 mins | Serving 4 | Difficulty: Easy)

Per serving: Cal: 200, Fat: 7g, Net Carbs: 1g, Protein: 34g

Ingredients

- Pork chops 4
- Salt 2 tsp
- Paprika 1 tsp
- Garlic powder 1 tsp
- Onion powder 1 tsp
- Oregano 1 tsp

Instructions

- ❖ Preheat the oven to 350 F (175 C).
- ❖ Clean and rinse the pork chops so the beef does not have extra water.
- ❖ To combine herbs and spices using a Ziplock container.
- ❖ Place one chop of pork in the zip lock bag at a time, seal, and shake until the chop of pork is thoroughly covered. Then put the pork chop on a wire rack over a parchment paper.
- ❖ Repeat the process with any chop of pork.
- ❖ Place them in the oven to bake them for 30 minutes.

Pork Chops with Cabbage Recipe

(Ready in about 12 mins | Serving 2 | Difficulty: Easy)

Per serving: Cal: 362, Fat: 21g, Net Carbs: 11g, Protein: 36g

Ingredients

- Pork chops 2
- Shredded cabbage 1/2
- Ghee 2 tbsp
- Tamari or coconut amino 1 tbsp
- Pepper ½ tsp
- Garlic powder ½ tsp

Instructions

- ❖ Heat the ghee over medium-high heat in a non-stick oven.
- ❖ When warm, add the pork chops and rub over the pepper and garlic powder. Stir in

the soy sauce. Fry for 4-5 mins on either side.

❖ When the second side of the chops is almost finished frying, add the cabbage to the grill.

❖ Cook for another 3 mins, constantly stirring until the cabbage is soft and faintly golden.

❖ Serve on a platter.

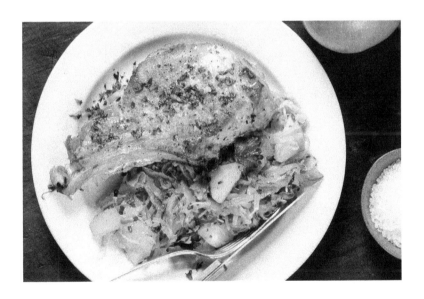

Crockpot Pork Chops - Keto

(Ready in about 3 hrs. 10 mins | Serving 4 | Difficulty: Medium)

Per serving: Cal: 283, Fat: 14g, Net Carbs: 3g, Protein: 35g

Ingredients

- Olive oil 2 tbsp
- Pork chops 4
- Large sliced onion 1
- Sliced mushrooms 1 cup
- Warm beef or chicken broth 1&1/2 cup
- Gluten-free tamari sauce 1 tbsp
- Salt & ground black pepper
- Chives

Instructions

- ❖ Heat the olive oil in a skillet and barbecue the pork chops until both sides are browned. Place separately.
- ❖ Fry the onions & mushrooms in the same sauce until they are caramelized. Deglaze the liquid over the pan and dump the liquid into the crockpot. Stir in the pork chops & cook on low for 3 hours. Remove the chops covered from the crockpot, season, & set aside to stay warm.
- ❖ Transfer the mixture of broth & onion into a clean pan, reduce to thick gravy. Drop the tamari, and then prepare the chops with the sauce.
- ❖ Complete with chives.

Keto Apples Dijon Pork Chop

(Ready in about 10 mins | Serving 2 | Difficulty: Easy)

Per serving: Cal: 560, Fat: 49g, Net Carbs: 2g, Protein: 34g

Ingredients

- Pork chops 2
- Ghee 4 tbsp
- Applesauce 2 tbsp
- Ghee 2 tbsp
- Dijon mustard 2 tbsp

- Salt & pepper>> to taste

Instructions

- ❖ In a wide pot, melt 4 Tbsp of ghee.
- ❖ Put chops of pork in. Place the chops of pork on its side using tongs, such that the fat cooks first in the ghee. Which makes it

brown & which renders a little of the fat. Then lie the pork chops, flat in the ghee, once the fat is a little crispy and browned.

❖ Cook them on either side for 3-4 mins. Check that the pork's internal temp exceeds 145 F (63 C) by using a meat thermometer. You can note it'll have a medium fresh pink inside while digging through the pork chops. If you like more cooked pork chops, just keep them in it for longer.

❖ In the meanwhile, blend well the applesauce, liquid ghee & mustard together.

❖ Serve the sauce with the pork chops and sprinkle with salt & pepper according to your taste.

Keto Bolognese Sauce and Spaghetti Squash

(Ready in about 45 mins | Serving 4 | Difficulty: Easy)

Per serving: Cal: 313, Fat: 19g, Net Carbs: 10g, Protein: 25g

Ingredients

- Spaghetti squash 1

- Ground or minced pork 1 lb.

- Can diced tomatoes 410 g

- Italian seasoning 2 tbsp

- Coconut or avocado oil to cook the meat with 2 tbsp

- Coconut or avocado oil to cook the spaghetti squash with 2 tbsp

- Salt & pepper>> to taste

- Chopped fresh parsley or basil ¼ cup

Instructions

- ❖ To 375 F, preheat the oven.
- ❖ Cut the spaghetti squash in 1/2 with caution (it can be hard to chop). Apply oil & salt on the squash's interior and put on a greased baking dish facing downwards.
- ❖ 45 mins bake (till the squash is soft). Let cool & use a fork to take out the spaghetti squash strands.
- ❖ Meanwhile, the meat sauce is cooked by pouring oil into a frying pan & brown the meat. Then add the chopped tomato and seasoning in Italian & let simmer until the squash is finished. Season to taste, with salt & pepper.
- ❖ Finally, just combine the meat sauce with the spaghetti squash or put the sauce on top of spaghetti squash & add parsley or basil to garnish with.

Low Cooker Ground Pork with Cauliflower Fried Rice

(Ready in about 6 hrs. | Serving 6 | Difficulty: Hard)

Per serving: Cal: 261, Fat: 11g, Net Carbs: 5g, Protein: 34g

Ingredients

Ingredients list for meat sauce:

- Medium diced onion 1/2
- Diced garlic cloves 3
- Ground pork 2 lbs.
- Tomato sauce or diced tomatoes ½ cup
- Italian seasoning 1 tbsp
- Bone broth ½ cup
- Salt & pepper>> to taste

Ingredients list for the cauliflower rice:

- Cauliflower 1
- Avocado oil 2 tbsp

- Carrot 1/2

- Salt & pepper>> to taste

Instructions

- ❖ Combine all the meat sauce ingredients to a slow cooker to make the meat sauce and set for 6 hours on low heat.
- ❖ To prepare the cauliflower rice, transfer the florets & carrots to the food processor, so convert to tiny rice-like bits. Squeeze out the maximum amount of extra oil.
- ❖ Apply avocado oil to a wide skillet & cook the cauliflower rice in batches until soft (approx. Ten minutes). Season to taste, with salt & black pepper.
- ❖ Ladle the cauliflower rice with the meat sauce and enjoy it. If needed, garnish with herbs such as chopped basil.

Keto Homemade Pork Sausage

(Ready in about 20 mins | Serving 4 | Difficulty: Easy)

Per serving: Cal: 202, Fat: 12g, Net Carbs: 1g, Protein: 24g

Ingredients

- Ground pork 1 lb.
- Garlic powder 1 tsp
- Onion powder 1 tsp
- Paprika 2 tsp
- Salt 1 tsp
- Cooking fat 2 tbsp

Instructions

❖ Mix ground pork with the onion powder, paprika, garlic powder, with salt in a clean bowl. Out of this meat mixture, use your hands to shape 8 little flat patties.

- ❖ Apply the cooking oil to the skillet & heat to low before adding in the patties.
- ❖ For the first side, let them cook for ten min before they get browned a little and turn them on the other side.
- ❖ Cook them for 7-8 mins on the second side before the meat's internal temp hits 145F.

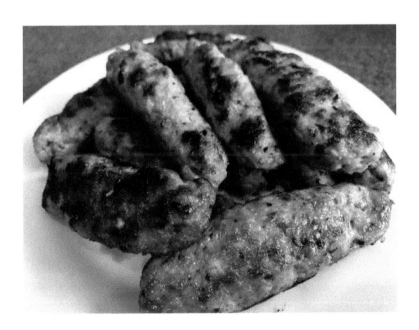

Asian-Flavored Pork Dumplings Pie

(Ready in about 20 mins | Serving 4 | Difficulty: Easy)

Per serving: Cal: 276, Fat: 21g, Net Carbs: 2g, Protein: 20g

Ingredients

For the filling:

- Ground pork ½ lb.
- Whisked egg 1
- Diced Chinese chives 1 c
- Diced garlic cloves 2
- Diced ginger 1 tsp
- Tamari sauce or coconut amino 2 tbsp
- Avocado oil 2 tbsp
- Salt >> to taste

For the egg wrap:

- Coconut oil 2 tbsp

- Whisked eggs 4

Instructions

❖ Mix all the filling ingredients in a bowl.

❖ In a separate bowl, whisk the eggs together.

❖ Add oil to a frying pan and make 2 thin egg pancakes with the whisked eggs. Place the first on a plate but leave the second in the frying pan but turn off the heat.

❖ In a separate frying pan, add in the avocado oil and then make a flat patty with the meat mixture and pan fry it. Flip the patty so that it's browned on both sides. Once the meat is cooked, place onto the egg pancake that's still in the frying pan. Place the other pancake on top and press down the egg pancakes' edges to seal them up.

❖ Cook for another 3-4 minutes, slice and serve.

Ground Pork Tacos

(Ready in about 25 mins | Serving 6 | Difficulty: Easy)

Per serving: Cal: 182, Fat: 9g, Net Carbs: 2g, Protein: 24g

Ingredients

- Avocado oil 2 tbsp
- Ground pork 1.5 lb.
- Diced medium onion 1/4
- Keto Egg Rolls Bowl

(Ready in about 15 mins | Serving 2 | Difficulty: Easy)

Per serving: Cal: 528, Fat: 33g, Net Carbs: 7g, Protein: 51g

Ingredients

- Avocado oil 3 tbsp
- Thin strips of ground pork or pork tenderloin 1 lb.
- Minced garlic cloves 2
- Sliced onion 1/2

- Sliced carrot 1/2
- Sliced Chinese cabbage 1/2
- Tamari soy sauce 2 tbsp
- Toasted sesame oil 1 tsp
- Chopped green onion 1

Instructions

- ❖ In a hot frying pan, apply the avocado oil & add in pork. Fry until light brown.
- ❖ Then substitute the onions, garlic, cabbage & carrot. Cook until tender.
- ❖ Add the sesame oil & tamari sauce.
- ❖ Garnish with green onions.

Keto Eggplant Burger

(Ready in about 20 mins | Serving 2 | Difficulty: Easy)

Per serving: Cal: 205, Fat: 5g, Net Carbs: 6g, Protein: 26g

Ingredients

For the eggplant burgers:

- Ground pork ½ lb.
- Japanese eggplants 1 lb.
- Diced green onions 2
- Minced ginger 1 tbsp
- Gluten-free tamari sauce or coconut amino 2 tbsp
- Salt 1 tsp
- Pinch of pepper

For the dipping sauce:

- Minced garlic cloves 4
- Gluten-free tamari sauce or coconut amino 4 tbsp

- Sesame oil 1 tsp

- Vinegar ½ tsp

Instructions

- ❖ Slice the eggplant into pieces 1 inch wide. Then create a slight cut into them to shape, still joined, "burger buns."
- ❖ Mix the ginger, green onions, tamari sauce, ground pork, salt, and black pepper. Place this combination of meat into the "buns."
- ❖ Steam it for 20 mins.
- ❖ Mix the tamari sauce, garlic, sesame oil, & vinegar in a little cup to produce the dipping sauce.
- ❖ Serve the eggplant burgers that have been cooked with dipping sauce.

Keto Asian Pork Ribs

(Ready in about 60 mins | Serving 4 | Difficulty: Medium)

Per serving: Cal: 505, Fat: 44g, Net Carbs: 1g, Protein: 25g

Ingredients

- Chopped pork spare ribs into individual ribs 2 lb.
- Fresh diced ginger 1 tbsp
- Diced green onions 2 tbsp
- Szechuan peppercorns ½ tbsp
- 2-star anise
- Diced garlic cloves 3
- Gluten-free tamari sauce or coconut amino 2 tbsp
- Avocado oil 2 tbsp
- Salt & pepper>> to taste

Instructions

- ❖ To a big pot of boiling water, add flour, Szechuan peppercorns, star anise, & ribs. Bring to boil, then cook until the meat is soft, for 45 mins. Skim away any shaping foam.
- ❖ Drain from the pot & remove ribs. Remove the star anise & peppercorns.
- ❖ Apply the avocado oil to the frying pan, then add the ginger and garlic. Put in ribs & cook on the medium-high fire. Add the coconut amino or tamari sauce, then season, to taste, with pepper and salt.
- ❖ Stir-fry ribs over high heat until fully covered and browned with the sauce.

Keto Slow Cooker Asian Pork's Rib

(Ready in about 3hrs. 20 mins | Serving 2 | Difficulty: Hard)

Per serving: Cal: 482, Fat: 38g, Net Carbs: 4g, Protein: 25g

Ingredients

- Baby back pork ribs 450g
- Sliced medium onion 1/2
- Garlic paste 1 tbsp
- Ginger paste 1 tbsp
- Chicken broth 1&1/2 c
- Gluten-free tamari sauce or coconut amino 2 tbsp
- Chinese five-spice seasoning ½ tsp
- Sliced green onions 2

Instructions

- ❖ Place the pork ribs rack inside the slow cooker. The rack may need to be halved to fit.
- ❖ Include the onions, paste for garlic, paste for the ginger, and broth for the meat. If the ribs are not completely coated, add up a little bit of broth until covered.
- ❖ Cover & cook for three hours at low flame.
- ❖ To keep warm, remove ribs & wrap in foil. Place this apart.
- ❖ Shift the onions & products from the slow cooker into the stove to a clean pan. Using a hand blender, blitz well (or use a food processor to blitz and move to the stove in the pan) and apply the Chinese 5-spice & tamari. Reduce the paste to dense and jammy over a relatively high flame.
- ❖ Taste the marinade and add in a bit of erythritol if you think it will improve from a little more sugar.
- ❖ Brush over the warm ribs with this marinade & garnish with onions.

Keto Baked Ribs Recipe

(Ready in about 3hrs. 5 mins | Serving 2 | Difficulty: Hard)

Per serving: Cal: 580, Fat: 51g, Net Carbs: 5g, Protein: 25g

Ingredients

- Baby back ribs 1 lb.
- Applesauce 2 tbsp
- Gluten-free tamari sauce or coconut amino 2 tbsp
- Olive oil 2 tbsp
- Fresh ginger 1 tbsp
- Garlic cloves 2
- Salt & pepper

Instructions

- ❖ Preheat the oven to 275 F (135 C) – change it to the minimum temperature if your oven does not go down to this point.
- ❖ Season with salt & pepper over ribs & cover securely with foil. Put the product onto a baking dish and bake in the oven for three hours at low temp.
- ❖ Mix olive oil, applesauce, tamari sauce, ginger, and garlic in a blender until it creates a purée.
- ❖ Take the ribs out from the oven after three hours, then adjust the heat in the oven up to 450 F (230 C) or just as high as the oven can go.
- ❖ With care, open the foil so the ribs can rest on top of the foil. Coat the ribs well with the marinade by using a brush. Put the ribs in the oven and bake for 5-10 mins until it becomes sticky with marinade.

Keto Fried Pork Tenderloin

(Ready in about 20 mins | Serving 2 | Difficulty: Easy)

Per serving: Cal: 389, Fat: 23g, Net Carbs: 0g, Protein: 47g

Ingredients

- Pork tenderloin 1 lb.
- Salt & pepper>> to taste
- Avocado or coconut oil 2 tbsp

Instructions

- ❖ Break the pork tenderloin into two-three pieces to fit more conveniently into your frying pan.
- ❖ Apply the oil to the frying pan & fry the pork tenderloin first on one side, using tongs. Using tongs, flip the pork tenderloin until that side is fried, then cook the other side until both sides are browned.

- ❖ Continue to turn the pork every several minutes until the meat thermometer displays just below 145F (63C), internal temperature. Since you remove it from the frying pan, the pork will begin to cook a little.
- ❖ Let the pork rest for a couple of minutes, then slice with a knife into one-inch-thick slices.

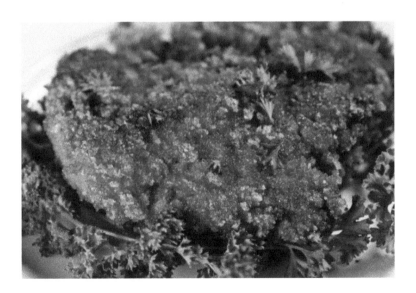

THANK YOU

Thank you for choosing *Ketogenic Diet: Salads and Pork Cookbook* for improving your cooking skills! I hope you enjoyed the recipes while making them and tasting them! If you're interested in learning new recipes and new meals to cook, go and check out the other books of the serie.